REAL FOOD FOR PREGNANCY BOOK

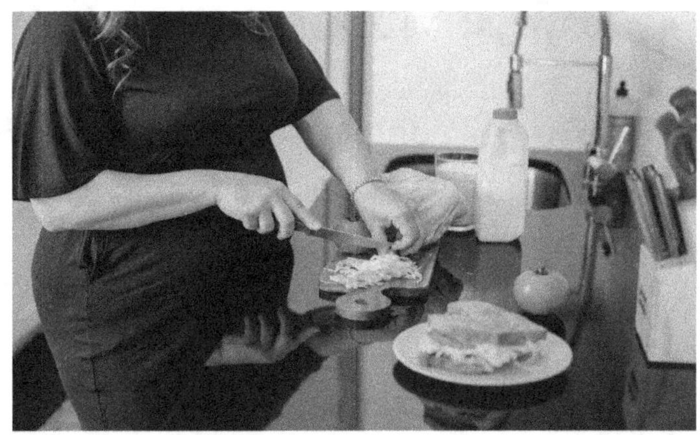

Nourishing Motherhood- "A Guide to Meal Planning for a Healthy and Vibrant Pregnancy Journey."

Yvonne Rose

TABLE OF CONTENTS

INTRODUCTION

Amidst a world flooded with processed temptations, a journey unfolds – one of nourishment, health, and the timeless bond between a mother and her unborn child. Meet Rose, a spirited soon-to-be-mother navigating the path of pregnancy. Her quest? Embracing real food's changing power for a radiant, blooming gestation.

In a whirlwind of conflicting advice and modern conveniences, She rediscovers the forgotten essence of wholesome, natural sustenance. From the vibrant colors of seasonal produce to the tender aroma of garden herbs, each morsel becomes a source to the life burgeoning within her. But her path isn't without challenges: societal norms, convenient alternatives, and cravings entice her towards shortcuts.

With unwavering determination, Rose unearths the hidden treasures of nourishing fare, guided by age-old wisdom and modern research. Through tantalizing recipes and nutrient-rich meals, she discovers a profound connection between her diet and her baby's well-being.

Journey alongside Rose as she reveals the profound impact of embracing real food during this sacred period. Experience the triumphs, the setbacks, and the invaluable lessons woven into this journey towards a healthy, vibrant pregnancy.

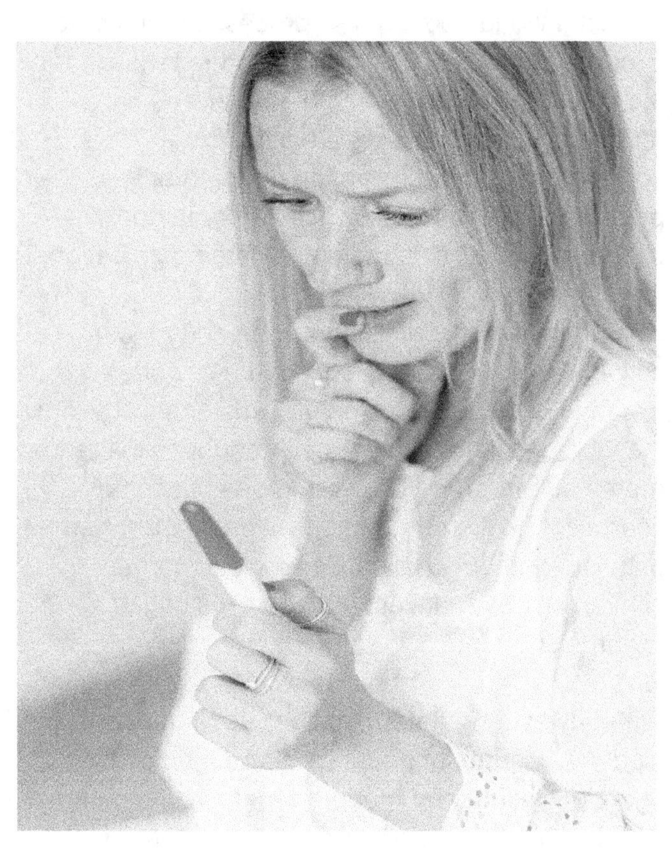

CHAPTER ONE

Understanding Pregnancy Nutrition

Pregnancy nutrition refers to the specific dietary needs and practices crucial for supporting the health and well-being of both the mother and the developing fetus during pregnancy. It involves understanding and meeting the increased nutritional requirements imposed by the physiological changes occurring within the pregnant woman's body and the demands of the growing baby

Key components of pregnancy nutrition

Macronutrients

These are the primary nutrients required in larger quantities, including carbohydrates, proteins, and fats. Carbohydrates serve as the main energy source, proteins aid in tissue growth and repair, and fats provide energy and aid in the development of the baby's brain and nervous system contributing to fetal development, preventing birth defects, supporting bone health, and ensuring a healthy immune system.

Hydration

Staying adequately hydrated is paramount during pregnancy. Water plays a vital role in transporting nutrients, aiding digestion, regulating body temperature, and supporting the amniotic fluid surrounding the baby.

Caloric Intake

While "eating for two" is a common misconception, pregnant women do need additional calories, but the exact amount varies depending on individual factors like pre-pregnancy weight, activity level, and trimester. It's more about the quality of calories rather than quantity, emphasizing nutrient-dense foods over empty calories.

Healthy Eating Pattern

Emphasizing a balanced diet that includes a variety of fruits, vegetables, whole grains, lean proteins, and healthy fats is crucial. Avoiding certain foods that pose risks, such as raw fish, unpasteurized dairy, and excessive caffeine, is also recommended.

Pregnancy nutrition is not just about individual nutrients but about creating a comprehensive dietary plan that considers the interplay of various elements to support the health and development of both mother and baby.

CHAPTER TWO

Nutritional meal plans and recipes for every trimester.

Making healthy meal and snack plans is essential because nutrition plays a big part in a happy and successful pregnancy. If you want to avoid morning sickness, sate cravings, maintain high energy, and fuel your body, you might want to make plans ahead of time, especially in the first trimester.

Is Nutrition important, why?

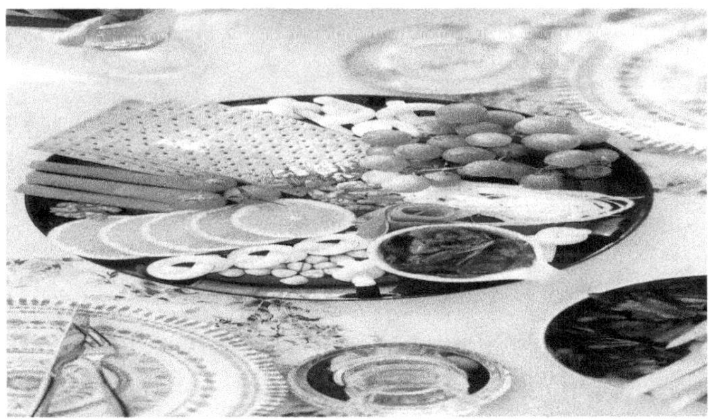

Since the fetus is still extremely little in the first trimester, you usually do not need any extra calories. To guarantee that the infant receives all the nutrients needed for healthy growth and development and that you are adequately fed, nutrition is still crucial.

At this point in your pregnancy, it is inaccurate to assume that you should eat twice as much food because you are **"eating for two."**

Some women will have morning sickness or nausea, which can occur at any time of the day despite the name), which might make them feel less hungry.

During the first trimester of pregnancy, it is best to follow a simple, nutrient-dense diet plan based on the **Dietary Guidelines for Americans,** which includes foods high in protein, whole grains, fruits, vegetables, and healthy fats. In addition, you will also need to be particularly aware of the following vitamins and minerals: **iron, calcium, vitamin D, folate, and choline.**

Iron aids in the delivery of oxygen to your fetus through red blood cells, while folate helps prevent birth abnormalities of the brain and spine.

Calcium and vitamin D contribute to normal bones, for both mom and baby.

Choline plays a role in your fetus's brain development and may also help prevent some common birth defects. Experts recommend that pregnant women get **450 mg of choline** each day.

Choline can be found in chicken, beef, eggs, milk, soy products, and peanuts. Although the body produces some choline on its own, it doesn't make enough to meet all your needs while you are pregnant. It's important to get choline from your diet because it is not found in most prenatal vitamins.

A healthcare provider can recommend the appropriate vitamin and mineral supplements during pregnancy, to ensure you get enough of these important nutrients (especially if you are unable to consume them in your diet).

Meal Planning

Meal planning is a proactive method of organizing and preparing meals in advance. It entails planning out your meals for a set length of time, usually a week or more. To expedite weekly cooking, this procedure includes selecting recipes, creating grocery lists, and prepping ingredients.

Components of meal planning

Recipe selection

This involves selecting recipes based on dietary choices, nutritional requirements, and the number of meals needed for the intended period.

Grocery list construction

It entails compiling a complete list of products required for the chosen recipes, ensuring that all necessary items are obtained in one trip to the shop.

Meal Preparation

To save time throughout the hectic week, prepare some meal components ahead of time, such as cutting vegetables, marinating proteins, or pre-cooking grains.

Scheduling

Allocating specific meals to specified days, considering circumstances like busy schedules or nights allotted for leftovers.

Advantages of meal planning

Time-saving:
Cooking on weekdays is shortened when ingredients or even entire meals are prepared in advance.

Encourages healthy eating
Makes it possible to make more deliberate decisions, guaranteeing a balanced nutrient intake and reducing reliance on junk food and fast food.

Minimizes food waste
It reduces food deterioration by making meals that utilize common components and only buying what is necessary.

Saves money: Buying ingredients in bulk or planning meals around items on sale helps cut costs and prevents unnecessary spending on impulse buying.

Overall, meal planning is a strategic approach to managing meals, providing structure, efficiency, and a healthier, more organized way of eating. Successful eating plans need to be individualized and holistic. Before starting a new diet plan, consult with a healthcare provider or a registered dietitian, especially if you have an underlying health condition.

Nutrition plays an important role in a healthy pregnancy, so planning for nutritious meals and snacks is paramount.
 Particularly in the **first trimester**, you may want to plan ahead to combat morning sickness, satisfy cravings, keep energy high, and nourish your body.

Meal planning can help keep you on track, no matter what your nutrition goal is.It plays a pivotal role throughout each trimester of pregnancy, ensuring both the mother and growing baby receive essential nutrients while addressing specific needs and challenges unique to each stage.

Effects of meal planning in each trimester

First trimester:
Meal planning in the initial phase focuses on combating morning sickness and addressing fatigue. It involves incorporating small, frequent meals rich in protein and complex carbohydrates. Planning for easily digestible foods like crackers, ginger tea, or small portions of lean proteins helps manage nausea. Additionally, ensuring an intake of folate-rich foods like leafy greens and citrus fruits aids in neural tube development.

Second trimester
This period often sees a decrease in morning sickness and a surge in energy. Meal planning now shifts towards increasing nutrient-dense foods to support the baby's rapid growth including calcium-rich foods like dairy products, iron from lean meats or legumes, and omega-3 fatty acids from fish supports bone development, red blood cell production, and brain development.

Third trimester
As the baby undergoes significant growth, meal planning becomes crucial for providing adequate energy and preparing for childbirth. emphasizing foods high in fiber, like whole grains and fruits, aids in digestion and prevents constipation common in

late pregnancy. Additionally, focusing on foods containing magnesium, such as nuts, seeds, and dark leafy greens, can help regulate blood pressure and reduce the risk of pre-eclampsia.

Meal planning also helps manage weight gain within healthy limits, ensuring a balanced intake of calories without excessive overeating. Moreover, it simplifies grocery shopping, cooking, and ensures a consistent intake of essential nutrients critical for both maternal and fetal health.
Overall, meal planning in every trimester serves as a compass, guiding expecting mothers to make informed food choices that support optimal health, energy levels, and fetal development throughout the transformative journey of pregnancy.

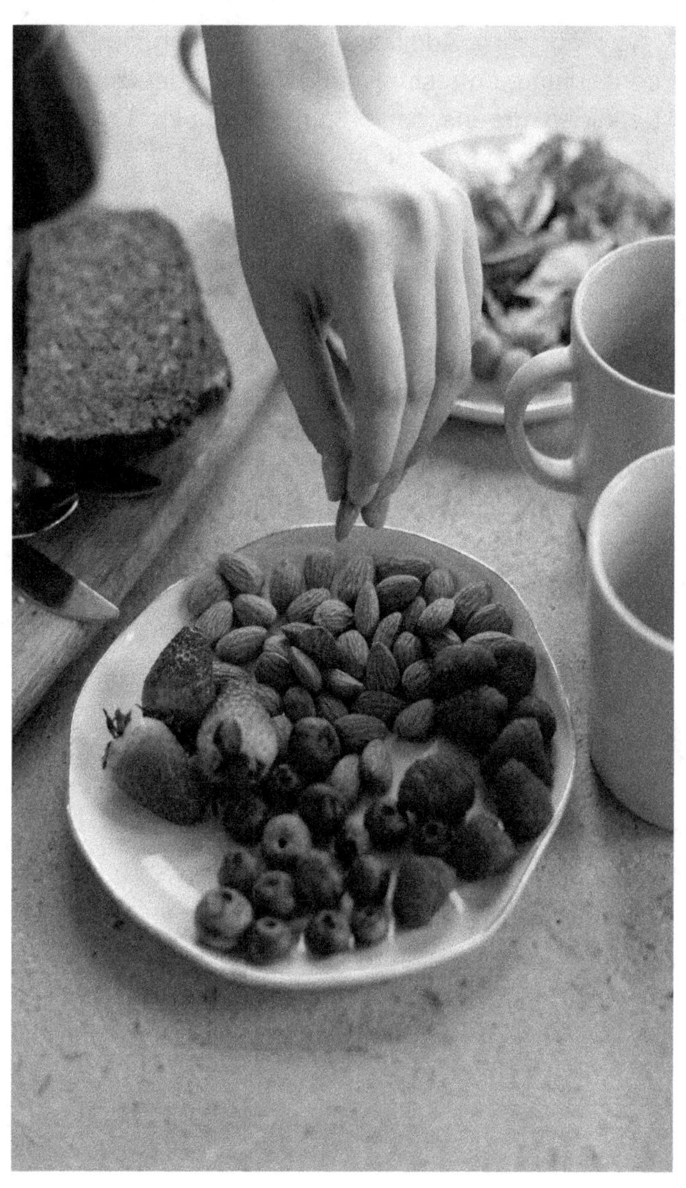

CHAPTER THREE

7-Day Sample Menu

This one-week meal plan was created for an individual with no dietary restrictions and a daily caloric need of roughly 2,000.
Nutrients including calcium, vitamin D, and folate are abundant in it. Your daily caloric target can change. Find out what it is below, and then modify the strategy to suit your needs. In order to more precisely assess and plan for your nutritional needs, think about consulting with a trained dietitian or visiting with a healthcare professional.

First trimester

 This diet plan consists of three meals and three snacks per day. It offers a decent ratio of protein, healthy fats, and carbohydrates—mostly from whole grains, vegetables, fruit, and legumes. It reflects the Dietary Guidelines for The section's American guidelines focus mainly on diet during pregnancy, particularly in the first trimester.

If you don't like certain dishes, feel free to **substitute** them with something you do, but try to keep within the same category. For example, you can replace one cup of rice with one cup of pasta. Consider substituting cauliflower for broccoli, but

keep cooking methods in mind (deep frying adds fat
and calories).

Breakfast.
One packet of plain oats mixed with two-thirds cup
of 2% milk.
One banana.
One tablespoon of walnuts
Micronutrients: 328 calories, 12 g protein, 55 g
carbohydrates, and 9 g fat.
Snack
1 cup edamame, shelled
1/4 avocado, chopped and sprinkled with lime juice
Micronutrients: 407 calories, 20 grams of protein,
27 grams of carbs, and 28 grams of fat.

Lunch
Two pieces whole grain bread with 3 ounces
canned light or skipjack tuna combined with 2
teaspoons mayonnaise and a one-ounce cheddar
cheese slice
1 cup spinach.
1 cup red pepper sticks.
Micronutrients: 470 calories, 40 grams protein, 43
grams carbs, and 17 grams of fat.

**"Because of the potential mercury
concentration, pregnant women should
exercise caution when consuming tuna"**.

Choose a brand that tests for mercury levels and select skipjack or canned light variants.

Snack
1/2 cup plain 2% Greek yogurt
1 cup strawberries
2 tablespoons granola
Micronutrients: 166 calories, 15 grams protein, 16 grams carbohydrates

Dinner
3 ounces grilled chicken
1 cup broccoli and 1 cup kale stir-fried in 2 teaspoons olive oil
1 cup pasta with 1/4 cup tomato sauce
Micronutrients: 501 calories, 39 grams protein, 59 grams carbohydrates, and 15 grams fat
Snack
1 medium apple.
One ounce cheddar cheese
Macronutrients: around 183 calories, 9 grams protein, 26 grams carbs, and 7 grams fat.
Daily totals: 2,055 calories, 135 grams of protein, 227 grams of carbs, and 81 grams of fat.

Day 2

Breakfast
Smoothie made with 3/4 cup plain 2% Greek yogurt, one banana, 2/3 cup 2% milk, and 1 tablespoon peanut butter.

Macronutrients: 452 calories, 27 grams protein, 45 grams carbs, and 20 grams of fat.
Snack
1 cup grapes.
2 tablespoons of almond butter.
Three whole grain crackers.
Macronutrients: 200 calories, 4 grams protein, 29 grams carbohydrates, and 10 grams of fat.

Lunch
Two pieces of whole grain bread, 2 hard-boiled eggs, and 2 tablespoons mayonnaise
1 cup spinach.
1 cup red pepper sticks.
Micronutrients: 442 calories, 24 grams protein, 43 grams carbs, and 21 grams of fat.
Snack
1/2 cup plain, 2% Greek yogurt.
1 cup strawberries.
2 tablespoons Granola
Micronutrients: 166 calories, 15 grams protein, 16 grams carbs, and 5 grams of fat.

Dinner
3 ounces grilled chicken.
Stir-fry 1 cup broccoli and 1 cup kale with 2 tablespoons of olive oil.
1 cup spaghetti and 1/4 cup tomato sauce.
Micronutrients: 501 calories, 39 g protein, 59 g carbs, and 15 g fat.
Snack
1 medium apple.

One ounce cheddar cheese
Macronutrients: around 183 calories, 9 grams protein, 26 grams carbs, and 7 grams fat.
Daily Totals: 2,055.

Day 3

Breakfast
1 cup of 2% plain Greek yogurt.
1 cup blueberries.
2 tablespoons of almond butter.
Macronutrients: 443 calories, 23 g protein, 34 g carbs, and 26 g fat
Snack
2 cups air popped popcorn
1 tablespoon of dark chocolate chips.
One spoonful of walnuts
Macronutrients: 184 calories, 4 g protein, 22 g carbs, and 10 g fat

Lunch
3 ounces grilled chicken.
2 cups of kale salad with 2 teaspoons olive oil vinaigrette and 1 tablespoon walnuts.
One tiny whole grain roll.
Macronutrients: 403 calories, 34 g protein, 33 g carbs, and 17 g fat
Snack
1/4 cup hummus.
1 cup carrot sticks.
2 tablespoons of mixed nuts.

Macronutrients: 235 calories, 10 g protein, 27 g carbs, and 20 g fat

Dinner
1 cup black beans
1 cup brown rice
1 cup diced red pepper
1 medium diced tomato
1/4 cup guacamole
Micronutrients: 578 calories, 23 grams protein, 102 grams carbohydrates, and 11 grams fat
Snack
One banana
1 tablespoon peanut butter
Micronutrients: 200 calories, 5 grams protein, 30 grams carbohydrates, and 8 grams fat
Daily Totals: 2,045 calories, 99 grams protein, 248 grams carbohydrates, and 92 grams fat

Day 4

Breakfast
Smoothie made with 3/4 cup plain 2% Greek yogurt, one banana, 2/3 cup 2% milk, and 1 tablespoon of peanut butter
Macronutrients: 452 calories, 27 grams protein, 45 grams carbohydrates, and 20 grams fat.
Snack
2 tablespoons almonds
2 tablespoons raisins
Micronutrients: 137 calories, 3 grams protein, 19 grams carbohydrates, and 8 grams fat.

Lunch
1 cup pasta mixed with 1/2 cup tomato sauce
3/4 cup cooked brown lentils
1 cup broccoli
1 tablespoon Parmesan cheese
Macronutrients: approximately 509 calories, 29 grams protein, 91 grams carbohydrates, and 6 grams fat.

Snack
2 tablespoons sunflower seeds
1 cup strawberries
Micronutrients: 152 calories, 4 grams protein, 16 grams carbohydrates, and 9 grams fat.

Dinner
3 ounces grilled trout (or any fish)
1 cup green beans
1 cup cooked brown rice
One small mixed green salad with 1 tablespoon olive oil and 1 1/2 teaspoons balsamic vinegar
Macronutrients: approximately 190 calories, 5 grams protein, 32 grams carbohydrates, and 6 grams fat
Daily Totals: 2,000 calories, 100 grams protein, 261 grams carbohydrates, and 72 grams fat.

Day 5

Breakfast
Two pieces of 100% whole wheat bread.
2 scrambled eggs cooked in 1 teaspoon butter.
One sliced tomato.

Macronutrients: 373 calories, 22g protein, 36g carbs, and 17g fat.

Snack

One orange

2 tablespoons of mixed nuts.

Macronutrients: 171 calories, 7 g protein, 29 g carbs, and 14 g fat.

Lunch

Combine 1 cup cooked pasta with 2 teaspoons pesto.

1 cup broccoli stir-fried with 1 teaspoon olive oil.

3 ounces grilled chicken contains 420 calories, 37 grams of protein, 43 grams of carbs, and 14 grams of fat.

Snack

1 ounce of cheddar cheese.

1 medium apple.

Macronutrients: 183 calories, 9g protein, 26g carbs, and 7g fat.

Dinner

Stir-fry 6 ounces of tofu with 1 teaspoon olive oil.

1 cup of cooked brown rice.

1 cup broccoli and 1 cup roasted cauliflower with 1 tablespoon olive oil.

Micronutrients:590 calories, 26 grams of protein, 62 grams of carbs, and 29 grams of fat.

Snack

1 cup strawberries.

1/2 cup vanilla ice cream.

1 tablespoon peanut butter.

Macronutrients: 334 calories, 7 grams protein, 38 grams carbs, and 19 grams of fat.
Daily totals are 2,071 calories, 108 grams of protein, 234 grams of carbs, and 100 grams of fat.

Day 6

Breakfast
3/4 cup plain, 2% Greek yogurt
1/4 cup granola.
1 cup strawberries.
Macronutrients include 368 calories, 20 grams of protein, 32 grams of carbs, and 17 grams of fat.
Snack
1 pear and 2 ounces Swiss cheese.
Micronutrients include 319 calories, 15 grams of protein, 31 grams of carbs, and 16 grams of fat.

Lunch
Two pieces of 100% whole wheat bread.
3.5 ounces canned salmon combined with 2 teaspoons mayonnaise.
1 medium tomato.
1 cup carrot sticks.
Micronutrients include 429 calories, 32 grams of protein, 54 grams of carbs, and 13 grams of fat.
Snack
Three wholegrain crackers.
2 tablespoons hummus.
1 cup carrot sticks.
Micronutrients: 160 calories, 5 g protein, 26 g carbs, and 6 g fat.

Dinner
1 cup lentils.
Combine 1 cup cooked pasta with 2 tablespoons olive oil and a few pinches of herbs and spices (oregano, cumin, etc.).
1 cup of diced red pepper.
1 medium chopped tomato.
2 tablespoons of guacamole.
Micronutrients include 572 calories, 28 grams of protein, 90 grams of carbs, and 15 grams of fat.
Snack
2 tablespoons sunflower seeds.
2 tablespoons of walnuts.
1 cup strawberries.
Micronutrients include 230 calories, 6 grams of protein, 18 grams of carbs, and 17 grams of fat.
Daily totals include 2,078 calories, 106 grams of protein, 251 grams of carbs, and 97 grams of fat.

Day 7:

Breakfast
1 cup of 2% plain Greek yogurt.
1 cup blueberries.
2 tablespoons of almond butter.
Macronutrients: 443 calories, 23g protein, 34g carbs, and 26g fat.
Snack
1 cup edamame, shelled
Micronutrients: 189 calories, 17 grams protein, 15 grams carbs, and 8 grams of fat.

Lunch:
Two pieces of 100% whole wheat bread, two hard-boiled eggs mashed with 2 teaspoons of mayonnaise.
1 medium tomato.
1 cup carrot sticks.
Micronutrients: 469 calories, 23 g protein, 54 g carbs, and 21 g fat.
Snack
1 medium apple.
1 ounce of cheddar cheese.
Three whole grain crackers.
Micronutrients include 243 calories, 10 grams of protein, 36 grams of carbs, and 10 grams of fat. 1 teaspoon balsamic vinegar.
2 tablespoons of guacamole.
Micronutrients include 544 calories, 35 grams of protein, 55 grams of carbs, and 20 grams of fat.
Snack
1 cup red pepper sticks.
1 cup of broccoli florets.
1/4 cup hummus.
Micronutrients: 160 calories, 8 g protein, 20 g carbs, and 6 g fat.
Daily Totals: 2,048 calories, 116 grams protein, 214 grams carbs, and 91 grams fat.

Healthy Meal Planning Tips during Pregnancy (First Trimester)

Savor seafood

Beneficial omega-3 fats found in fatty fish like salmon and trout aid in the development of a baby's brain.

Nonetheless, mercury can be harmful to a developing fetus and is present in certain types of fish. Steer clear of orange roughy, marlin, shark, swordfish, tilefish, bigeye tuna, and king mackerel. Just six ounces of white (albacore) tuna should be consumed each week. Select lighter or skipjack tuna, as it has less mercury.

Carry some bland meals on hand

Try some bland toast, crackers, bananas, or applesauce if you feel queasy. Aiming for multiple modest meals throughout the day rather than one large one may also be helpful.

Eat less fattening meals, such as deep-fried or greasy foods, as these can cause nausea and further delay the emptying of the stomach.

For choline, add eggs

A healthy pregnancy requires choline. Meat, beans, lentils, and egg yolks are good sources. Your prenatal supplement might not contain choline, so it's crucial to obtain it from a diet. Ask your healthcare practitioner if you need a choline supplement, especially if you avoid eggs (which are the best nutritional source of choline).

Pick your milk substitutes wisely

Make sure plant-based milk substitutes are supplemented with calcium and vitamin D if you want to forgo cow's milk. Because the calcium fortification settles to the bottom as sediment, make sure to give the beverage container a good shake before adding liquid. Research revealed that compared to well-mixed samples, unshaken almond and soy samples had 14 and 18% lower calcium levels; The calcium concentrations of the unshaken rice and oat samples were 96.7 and 96% lower than those of the well-mixed samples.

"Morning sickness may prevent you from consuming a wide variety of foods during the first trimester, so you may need to postpone meal planning and stick to things like simple carbohydrates. When feasible, strive to include foods that are high in nutrients, even though this can be difficult. During this stage, foods like bread, crackers, dry cereal, and rice could be easier to tolerate".

2nd trimester

In the second trimester, morning sickness is usually halted as the body is familiar with all the developmental processes coupled with hormone release. Meal plans during this time should be majored on providing energy and adequate nutrition for the mother and baby. To follow these samples, here is a basic, intelligible meal plan with back-up rationales on "what" and "why".

Day 1

Breakfast:
Spinach and feta omelet on whole grain toast.
Lunch:
Quinoa salad with grilled chicken, mixed veggies, and citrus vinaigrette.
Dinner:
Baked salmon filled with roasted sweet potatoes and steamed broccoli.
Rationelle:
The spinach in the omelet supplies folate, which is required for neural tube development. Quinoa provides a complete protein supply, while salmon contains omega-3 fatty acids that are essential for brain and vision development in the fetus.

Day 2:

Breakfast
Greek yogurt parfait with mixed berries and chia seeds.

Lunch:
 Lentil soup with whole grain bread and mixed greens salad.
Dinner:
Turkey meatballs with whole wheat spaghetti, marinara sauce, and sautéed spinach.

Rationelle

Greek yogurt contains calcium and probiotics that promote bone health and digestion. Lentils are high in iron, which is vital for preventing anemia, whereas whole grains provide fiber, which is good for digestion.

Breakfast:

Whole grain bread with avocado mash and poached eggs.

Lunch:

Grilled vegetable and hummus wrap with a side of mixed fruits.

Dinner:

Stir-fried tofu with brown rice and mixed vegetables.

Rationelle:

Avocado delivers healthful fats, tofu gives plant-based protein, and brown rice provides energy with a low glycemic index, which promotes blood sugar stability.

Breakfast

Overnight oats with almond milk, banana slices, and cinnamon.

Lunch

Quinoa-stuffed bell peppers served with mixed greens.

Dinner:

Baked chicken breast, roasted Brussels sprouts, and quinoa pilaf.

Rationelle:

Oats provide fiber and long-lasting energy. Bell peppers include vitamin C, which aids iron absorption from quinoa, whole chicken provides protein and iron.

Day 5:

Breakfast:

Whole grain pancakes topped with fresh berries and Greek yogurt.

Lunch:

Tuna salad sandwich with whole grain bread and carrot sticks.

Dinner:

Grilled shrimp skewers with zucchini and couscous.

Rationelle:

Berries give antioxidants, whole grains supply complex carbs, and shrimp provide protein and omega-3 fatty acids that are essential for embryonic development.

Day 6:

Breakfast

Avocado toast with poached eggs and a side of mixed berries.

Lunch:

Quinoa salad with grilled chicken, mixed veggies, and citrus vinaigrette.

Dinner
Stir-fried tofu with brown rice and mixed vegetables.

Rationelle:
Avocado provides healthful fats and folate, while quinoa contains full protein. Tofu contains plant-based protein and a variety of vital elements.

Day 7

Breakfast
Smoothie with spinach, banana, almond milk, and protein powder.

Lunch
Caprese salad with tomatoes, mozzarella, basil, and a splash of balsamic glaze.

Dinner
Baked cod with roasted asparagus and quinoa.

Rationelle
The smoothie has folate from spinach, while cod contains protein and vitamin D, both of which are essential for bone formation. Caprese salad provides calcium and healthy fats.

This meal plan incorporates a variety of nutrient-dense foods, including lean proteins, whole grains, healthy fats, and a plethora of fruits and vegetables, ensuring a well-rounded intake of essential nutrients vital for both maternal health and fetal development during the second trimester.

Third trimester

During the third trimester, carbohydrate intake is reduced and replaced with foods high in protein, iron, folate, and other nutrients.

This is to promote the complete development of the baby's exterior and internal structures while also preparing the mother's body for labor and delivery. The food samples listed below can be used as a guide at this stage.

Day 1:

Breakfast
Whole grain cereal topped with sliced bananas and almonds.

Lunch
Chickpea salad with mixed greens, tomatoes, cucumbers, and tahini dressing.

Dinner
Grilled chicken breast with roasted sweet potatoes and steaming green beans.

Rationelle
Whole grain cereal gives both fiber and energy. Chickpeas contain protein and folate, whereas chicken has lean protein and iron, which aids with blood synthesis and fetal growth.

Breakfast

Spinach and cheese omelet served with whole grain toast.

Lunch

Quinoa-stuffed bell peppers served with mixed greens.

Dinner

Baked salmon with sauteed spinach and quinoa pilaf.

Rationelle

The spinach in the omelet contains folate, while the salmon has omega-3 fatty acids, which are essential for brain development. Quinoa has all of the essential protein components.

Day 3

Breakfast

Greek yogurt parfait with mixed berries and granola.

Lunch

Lentil soup with whole grain bread and a mixed green salad.

Dinner:

Turkey meatballs with whole wheat spaghetti and marinara sauce, topped with roasted vegetables.

Rationelle

Greek yogurt contains calcium and probiotics, whereas lentils supply iron and fiber. Whole wheat pasta contains complex carbs, which provide long-term energy.

Day 4:

Breakfast
Whole grain pancakes with fresh fruit and a dollop of Greek yogurt.
Lunch
Tuna salad sandwich on whole grain bread with a side of carrot sticks.
Dinner
Grilled shrimp skewers with quinoa and roasted Brussels sprouts.
Rationelle
Whole grain pancakes provide energy, while tuna supplies protein and omega-3 fatty acids. Shrimp offers protein and other essential nutrients.

Day 5:

Breakfast
Overnight oats with almond milk, sliced bananas, and a sprinkle of cinnamon.
Lunch
Veggie and hummus wrap with a side of mixed fruit.
Dinner
Baked chicken with roasted vegetables and brown rice.

Rationelle

Overnight oats provide fiber and sustained energy. Hummus offers plant-based protein, and chicken provides lean protein and essential nutrients.

Day 6

Breakfast

Avocado toast with poached eggs and a side of mixed berries.

Lunch

Quinoa salad with grilled chicken, mixed vegetables, and a citrus vinaigrette.

Dinner

Stir-fried tofu with brown rice and assorted vegetables.

Rationelle

Avocado supplies healthy fats and folate, while quinoa offers complete protein. Tofu provides plant-based protein and various essential nutrients.

Day 7

Breakfast

Smoothie with spinach, banana, almond milk, and a scoop of protein powder.

Lunch

Caprese salad with tomatoes, mozzarella, basil, and a drizzle of balsamic glaze.

Dinner

Baked cod with roasted asparagus and quinoa.

Rationelle

Spinach in the smoothie provides folate, while cod offers protein and vitamin D crucial for bone development. Caprese salad supplies calcium and healthy fats.

The emphasis of this meal plan is on nutrient-dense foods, which include whole grains, lean meats, healthy fats, and an assortment of fruits and vegetables. It attempts to supply vital nutrients—like iron, calcium, protein, and omega-3 fatty acids—that are needed during the third trimester in order to support the health and growth of the fetus during this crucial phase of pregnancy.

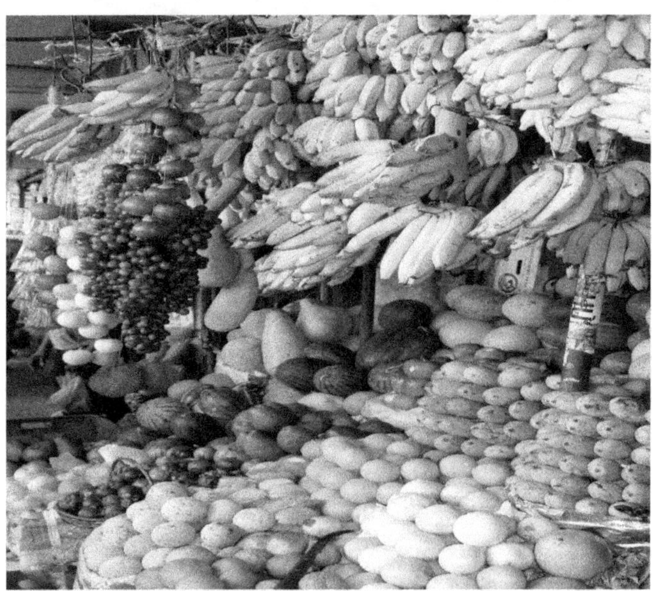

CHAPTER FOUR

Using Nutrition to Address Common Pregnancy Concerns

How can your diet become a magic potion that relieves pregnancy fatigue, heartburn, and morning sickness? Discover the amazing world where ordinary foods can become magical weapons that assist women overcome common pregnancy anxieties. Find out how having a healthy dinner might help you have a more comfortable and energetic pregnancy.

Rose was trapped in the "**Cloud of Morning Sickness,**" a confusing fog that interrupted her peaceful days. She learnt from the "**Real Food for Pregnancy Book**" that eating crackers, drinking ginger tea, and eating small, frequent meals with apples or bananas helped settle her tummy. These simple, light dishes calmed the storm in her stomach, allowing her to greet each sunrise with renewed vitality.

The Veil of Fatigue:

As Rose continued on her quest, she came across the "Veil of Fatigue," a malaise that cast shadows over her sunny days. With the Sage's guidance, she adopted a diet rich in whole grains like oats and brown rice, lean proteins like chicken and beans, and greens like spinach and kale.

The Fire of Heartburn:
During her wanderings, Rose encountered the
"Fire of Heartburn," a burning discomfort that
disturbed her tranquility. Following the Sage's
advice, she changed her diet, eschewing spicy or
acidic foods in favor of oatmeal, bananas, and
almonds. These soft foods extinguished the flames,
providing relief from the blistering heat.

The Riddle of Cravings:
Rose experienced the "Riddle of Cravings," a
whimsical need for specific delicacies that disrupted
her balance. Understanding her desires as signals
for nutrition, she ate a spectrum of foods, including
fruits, vegetables, and whole grains. Crafting
nutritional alternatives to her cravings pleased her
taste senses while also providing critical nutrients
for her and her baby's health.

The Twilight of Insomnia:
As the stars twinkled above, Rose grappled with
the "Twilight of Insomnia," finding rest elusive.
Guided by the Sage's advice, she sipped herbal
teas, indulged in almonds and yogurt before
bedtime, and practiced relaxation techniques.
These simple rituals eased her into slumber,
offering respite from sleepless nights.

In Expectara, Rose learnt that nurturing her body
with simple, nutrient-rich foods was the magical
wand that combated these pregnancy concerns.
Every obstacle she overcame revealed the strength
of the food, giving her the means to traverse the
magical but turbulent voyage.

CHAPTER FIVE

Mindful Eating and Wellness Practices for Expecting Moms.

In the grand narrative of pregnancy, where each chapter tells a tale of new beginnings, a curious question emerges: Why do some expecting mothers miss the magic of mindful eating and wellness practices? Amidst the whirlwind of cravings and the daily hustle, are the secrets to feeling good and nourished overlooked? Imagine if choosing food became a treasure hunt for joy and vitality, and moments of calmness and well-being became everyday companions. Why do some moms-to-be unintentionally bypass these tools that could infuse this wondrous journey with grace and strength? Could the bustling busyness of preparation overshadow the importance of tending to one's body and spirit during this extraordinary passage? Let's embark on a journey to uncover why some expecting mothers may inadvertently miss the opportunity to embrace the transformative potential of mindful eating and holistic wellness, nurturing not only themselves but also their blossoming miracles.

Mindful eating and wellness practices are invaluable tools for expecting mothers, offering a holistic approach to nurturing both the body and mind during pregnancy.

Mindful Eating

Mindful eating is a practice that involves paying full attention to the present moment while consuming food. It encompasses awareness of sensations, thoughts, and emotions associated with eating. For expecting moms, mindful eating is about fostering a deeper connection between food, body, and overall well-being. Its components are explained below.

Sensory Awareness

It involves engaging all the senses while eating, savoring the colors, textures, flavors, and aromas of food. For expecting mothers, this means appreciating the nourishment and vitality each bite offers, making the dining experience more gratifying.

Present-Moment Awareness

Mindful eating encourages being fully present without distractions, such as phones or television, during meals. This practice helps expecting moms focus on their body's cues, recognizing hunger and satiety signals, ensuring they eat in response to genuine physical needs.

Non-judgmental Observation

It encourages a non-critical, non-judgmental attitude towards food choices and eating habits. Expecting moms can explore their food preferences without guilt, cultivating a positive relationship with food during this transformative period.

Emotional Awareness

Mindful eating involves acknowledging emotions that arise during eating, such as stress or happiness. For expecting moms, this practice helps in recognizing emotional triggers related to food, allowing for more conscious and intentional choices.

Gratitude and Appreciation:

Cultivating gratitude for the food on the plate, its source, and the efforts behind it is a key aspect of mindful eating. This practice helps expecting moms appreciate the nourishment they provide themselves and their growing baby.

Wellness Practices for Expecting Moms:

Regular Physical Activity

Safe and moderate exercise tailored to pregnancy helps maintain overall fitness, manage weight, and improve mood. Activities like prenatal yoga, swimming, or walking promote flexibility, strength, and relaxation.

Adequate Rest and Sleep

Prioritizing adequate rest is crucial for expecting moms. Quality sleep supports physical health and emotional well-being, aiding in the body's recovery and reducing stress.

Stress Management Techniques

Practicing relaxation techniques such as deep breathing, meditation, or prenatal massage helps reduce stress levels. Lowering stress positively impacts both maternal and fetal health.

Balanced Nutrition

 A well-rounded diet rich in fruits, vegetables, whole grains, lean proteins, and healthy fats provides essential nutrients crucial for fetal development and maternal health. Mindful eating practices can enhance the experience of nourishing the body with wholesome foods.

Hydration

Staying adequately hydrated is essential. Water supports the body's functions, aids digestion, prevents dehydration, and maintains amniotic fluid levels.

Prenatal Care and Check-ups

Regular visits to healthcare providers ensure the monitoring of both the mother's and baby's health, addressing any concerns promptly.

In summary, mindful eating encourages a deepened relationship with food, promoting conscious choices and a positive eating experience for expecting moms. Coupled with holistic wellness practices encompassing physical activity, rest, stress management, balanced nutrition, and regular prenatal care, these approaches nurture the body and mind, fostering optimal health and well-being throughout the journey of pregnancy.

IMPORTANCE OF MINDFUL EATING AND WELLNESS PRACTICES

Mindful eating and wellness practices play pivotal roles in fostering a healthy pregnancy by nurturing both the physical and emotional well-being of expecting mothers. Here are some solid importances:

Optimal Nutrient Intake:
 Mindful eating ensures a well-balanced diet, providing essential nutrients crucial for fetal development and maternal health. This practice supports the body's increased nutritional needs during pregnancy, promoting a healthier environment for the baby's growth.

Weight Management
Mindful eating aids in maintaining a healthy weight during pregnancy. It encourages listening to the body's hunger and fullness cues, preventing

excessive weight gain while ensuring adequate
nourishment for both the mother and baby.

Stress Reduction

Wellness practices like meditation, deep breathing,
and relaxation techniques alleviate stress and
anxiety levels. Lowering stress is vital for a
healthier pregnancy, reducing the risk of
complications and positively impacting the baby's
development.

Enhanced Digestion

Mindful eating involves chewing food slowly and
being present while consuming meals. This practice
aids digestion, minimizing digestive discomforts like
bloating or indigestion commonly experienced
during pregnancy.

Improved Sleep Quality

Engaging in wellness practices promotes better
sleep. Quality sleep is crucial for expecting mothers
as it supports physical health, reduces fatigue, and
contributes to overall well-being.

Emotional Balance

Mindful eating and wellness practices encourage
emotional awareness and resilience. They help
manage mood swings, promoting a more stable
emotional state during the ups and downs of
pregnancy.

Bonding Experience

Mindful eating can turn mealtime into a nurturing and bonding experience with the baby. It fosters a deeper connection between the mother and her growing child, enhancing the overall pregnancy experience.

Preparation for Labor
Engaging in wellness practices like prenatal yoga or exercises prepares the body for labor and delivery. These practices improve flexibility, strength, and relaxation techniques, aiding in a smoother birthing experience.

In essence, practicing mindful eating and wellness techniques during pregnancy is not just about physical health; it's a holistic approach that nurtures the mind, body, and spirit. These practices contribute significantly to a healthier pregnancy journey, positively impacting both the mother and the developing baby.

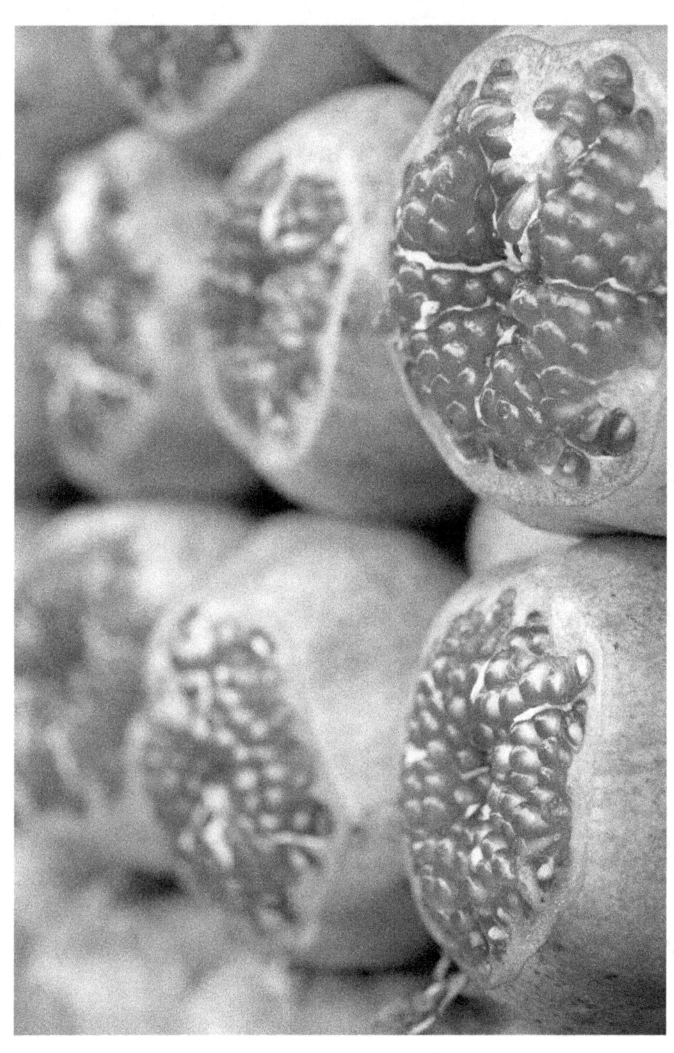

CHAPTER SIX

Practical Tips for a Real Food Lifestyle Beyond Pregnancy

Transitioning to a real food lifestyle beyond pregnancy is a wonderful continuation of the nourishing habits developed during this transformative period. Here are some practical tips to embrace this approach:

Focus on Whole Foods

Prioritize whole, unprocessed foods such as fruits, vegetables, whole grains, lean proteins, and healthy fats. Opt for foods as close to their natural state as possible, minimizing the intake of processed and refined products.

Read Labels Mindfully

When purchasing packaged foods, read labels attentively. Choose products with fewer ingredients, avoiding artificial additives, preservatives, and excessive sugar or sodium content.

Plan and Prepare Meals

Meal planning is key to maintaining a real food lifestyle. Allocate time for planning meals, creating grocery lists, and prepping ingredients in advance.

This approach simplifies cooking and encourages healthier choices.

Cook at Home

Cooking meals at home allows better control over ingredients and portions. Experiment with various recipes using fresh produce, herbs, and spices to enhance flavors without relying on processed seasonings.

Prioritize Seasonal and Local Produce

Embrace seasonal fruits and vegetables as they tend to be fresher, more flavorful, and nutrient-dense. Support local farmers' markets or community-supported agriculture (CSA) for fresh, locally sourced produce.

Include a Variety of Foods

Incorporate a diverse range of foods to ensure a broad spectrum of nutrients. Rotate through different vegetables, grains, proteins, and fats to achieve a balanced and varied diet.

Choose Healthy Fats

Opt for healthy fats like avocados, nuts, seeds, olive oil, and fatty fish rich in omega-3 fatty acids. Heart health and general well-being are supported by these lipids.

Mindful Eating Practices

Practice mindful eating by savoring each bite, chewing slowly, and being present during meals. This habit encourages better digestion, aids in portion control, and fosters a deeper connection with food.

Stay Hydrated

Water is essential for overall health. Aim to drink adequate water throughout the day, and consider herbal teas or infused water for variety and added nutrients.

Follow Your Body's Cues:

Pay attention to your body's indicators of hunger and fullness. Eat when hungry and stop when satisfied, avoiding overeating.

Minimize Sugary Beverages and Snacks

Limit intake of sugary drinks and processed snacks. Instead, opt for healthier alternatives like homemade smoothies, fruit, nuts, or yogurt.

Moderation is Key

Embrace balance and moderation in your food choices. Allow occasional treats or indulgences without guilt, while maintaining a primarily real food-based diet.

Learn and Adapt

Continuously educate yourself about nutrition and real food options. Be flexible and adaptable, making adjustments based on personal preferences and lifestyle changes.

Embracing a real food lifestyle beyond pregnancy isn't just a temporary diet but a sustainable approach to nourishing your body and maintaining optimal health. By incorporating these practical tips into daily life, you'll foster long-term habits that support vitality, energy, and overall well-being for years to come.

CONCLUSION

As you embark on the miraculous journey of pregnancy, remember that the power of real food is not merely sustenance—it's an elixir that breathes life into every moment of this celestial passage. It's the vibrant canvas upon which your baby's future health is painted, the gentle whisper that nurtures your soul, and the unwavering embrace that supports you through every heartbeat of this remarkable journey.

Real food isn't just about nutrients; it's about the symphony of flavors dancing on your palate, the colors of fresh produce painting a masterpiece on your plate, and the aroma of wholesome meals weaving stories of nourishment and vitality. It's the embodiment of love—love for your growing miracle, love for your own body, and love for the journey you're courageously traversing.

As you savor the crispness of an apple, the richness of leafy greens, or the tenderness of a home-cooked meal, know that you're creating a sanctuary of well-being for you and your baby. With each mindful bite, you're infusing vitality into your pregnancy, crafting a tapestry of health that transcends the realm of mere existence and embraces the essence of vibrant living.

The journey empowered by real food isn't just a chapter; it's a legacy—a legacy of health, resilience, and boundless love. It's the legacy you leave imprinted in every heartbeat, every gentle kick, and every radiant smile shared between you and your little one. It's the legacy of a journey sculpted with grace, nourishment, and the profound magic of real, wholesome nourishment.

So, let the magic of real food be your guiding light, your comforting embrace, and your unwavering ally as you journey through this sacred time. Embrace its power, cherish its essence, and witness the awe-inspiring transformation it weaves into your pregnancy, leaving you in absolute wonder at the miracles it bestows upon your remarkable journey of motherhood.

DAILY MEAL PLAN REMARKS

DAY	MEAL	REMARK